100 Questions & Answers About Depression

by Laura L. Smith, PhD

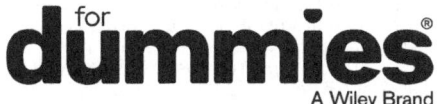

100 Questions & Answers About Depression For Dummies®

Published by: **John Wiley & Sons, Inc.**, 111 River Street, Hoboken, NJ 07030-5774, www.wiley.com

Copyright © 2026 by John Wiley & Sons, Inc. All rights reserved, including rights for text and data mining and training of artificial technologies or similar technologies.

No part of this publication may be reproduced, stored in a retrieval system or transmitted in any form or by any means, electronic, mechanical, photocopying, recording, scanning or otherwise, except as permitted under Sections 107 or 108 of the 1976 United States Copyright Act, without the prior written permission of the Publisher or authorization through payment of the appropriate per-copy fee to the Copyright Clearance Center, Inc., 222 Rosewood Drive, Danvers, MA 01923, (978) 750-8400, fax (978) 750-4470, or on the web at www.copyright.com. Requests to the Publisher for permission should be addressed to the Permissions Department, John Wiley & Sons, Inc., 111 River Street, Hoboken, NJ 07030, (201) 748-6011, fax (201) 748-6008, or online at http://www.wiley.com/go/permissions.

The manufacturer's authorized representative according to the EU General Product Safety Regulation is Wiley-VCH GmbH, Boschstr. 12, 69469 Weinheim, Germany, e-mail: Product_Safety@wiley.com.

Trademarks: Wiley, For Dummies, the Dummies Man logo, Dummies.com, Making Everything Easier, and related trade dress are trademarks or registered trademarks of John Wiley & Sons, Inc. and may not be used without written permission. All other trademarks are the property of their respective owners. John Wiley & Sons, Inc. is not associated with any product or vendor mentioned in this book.

LIMIT OF LIABILITY/DISCLAIMER OF WARRANTY: THE CONTENTS OF THIS WORK ARE INTENDED TO FURTHER GENERAL SCIENTIFIC RESEARCH, UNDERSTANDING, AND DISCUSSION ONLY AND ARE NOT INTENDED AND SHOULD NOT BE RELIED UPON AS RECOMMENDING OR PROMOTING A SPECIFIC METHOD, DIAGNOSIS, OR TREATMENT BY PHYSICIANS FOR ANY PARTICULAR PATIENT. THE PUBLISHER AND THE AUTHOR MAKE NO REPRESENTATIONS OR WARRANTIES WITH RESPECT TO THE ACCURACY OR COMPLETENESS OF THE CONTENTS OF THIS WORK AND SPECIFICALLY DISCLAIM ALL WARRANTIES, INCLUDING WITHOUT LIMITATION ANY IMPLIED WARRANTIES OF FITNESS FOR A PARTICULAR PURPOSE. CERTAIN AI SYSTEMS HAVE BEEN USED IN THE CREATION OF THIS WORK. IN VIEW OF ONGOING RESEARCH, EQUIPMENT MODIFICATIONS, CHANGES IN GOVERNMENTAL REGULATIONS, AND THE CONSTANT FLOW OF INFORMATION RELATING TO THE USE OF MEDICINES, EQUIPMENT, AND DEVICES, THE READER IS URGED TO REVIEW AND EVALUATE THE INFORMATION PROVIDED IN THE PACKAGE INSERT OR INSTRUCTIONS FOR EACH MEDICINE, EQUIPMENT, OR DEVICE FOR, AMONG OTHER THINGS, ANY CHANGES IN THE INSTRUCTIONS OR INDICATION OF USAGE AND FOR ADDED WARNINGS AND PRECAUTIONS. READERS SHOULD CONSULT WITH A SPECIALIST WHERE APPROPRIATE. NO WARRANTY MAY BE CREATED OR EXTENDED BY ANY PROMOTIONAL STATEMENTS. NEITHER THE PUBLISHER NOR THE AUTHOR SHALL BE LIABLE FOR ANY DAMAGES ARISING THEREFROM.

For general information on our other products and services, please contact our Customer Care Department within the U.S. at 877-762-2974, outside the U.S. at 317-572-3993, or fax 317-572-4002. For technical support, please visit https://hub.wiley.com/community/support/dummies.

Wiley publishes in a variety of print and electronic formats and by print-on-demand. Some material included with standard print versions of this book may not be included in e-books or in print-on-demand. If this book refers to media that is not included in the version you purchased, you may download this material at http://booksupport.wiley.com. For more information about Wiley products, visit www.wiley.com.

Library of Congress Control Number is available from the publisher.

ISBN 978-1-394-36873-0 (pbk); ISBN 978-1-394-36875-4 (ebk); ISBN 978-1-394-36874-7 (ebk)

Contents at a Glance

Table of Contents

Introduction

I n the United States, depression is one of the more common mental health disorders. According to the Centers for Disease Control and Prevention (CDC), in 2024, 5 percent of American adults "regularly reported feelings of depression," and in 2023, 40 percent of American high school students experienced symptoms of depression. I wrote this book to answer common questions about depression — what it is, what causes it, how it differs from everyday sadness, and the treatment options available.

About This Book

This book is a reference, which means you don't need to read the chapters in order from beginning to end and you don't have to remember anything — there isn't a test at the end of it.

Within this book, you may note that some web addresses break across two lines of text. If you're reading this book in print and want to visit one of these web pages, simply key in the web address exactly as it's noted in the text, pretending as though the line break doesn't exist. If you're reading this as an e-book, you've got it easy — just click the web address to be taken directly to the web page.

Foolish Assumptions

In writing this book, I made just a couple of assumptions about you, the reader:

» You have depression or know someone who has depression.

» You have questions, and you want answers.

If those basic assumptions apply to you, you've come to the right place.

Icon Used in This Book

This book uses the following icon in the margins:

TIP

When you see the Tip icon, you'll find information that will make your life a little easier, at least when it comes to depression.

Where to Go from Here

If you aren't sure where to begin, head to the Table of Contents and skim through the questions until you find one that catches your eye. Or, if you have a specific topic in mind, search for it in the Index. Want to know absolutely everything? Turn the page and start in with Part 1.

1

Understanding Depression

This part explains what depression is, the biology behind depression, what causes depression, and the risk factors for developing it. If you or someone you love has recently received a diagnosis of depression, this part is for you.

DID YOU KNOW?

A common myth about depression is that people should just deal with their problems and get over themselves. Not true at all. Depression is a mental health disorder, not a symptom of weakness.

Chapter **1**

Understanding Depression

From that Sunday blues feeling that many people experience before beginning the workweek, to literally being unable to get out of bed, depression has a big tent. This chapter describes symptoms and types of depression, as well as how depression differs from other mental health disorders.

What Is Depression?

Depression is a mental health condition that includes persistent feelings of sadness and beliefs that the future is hopeless and that life is joyless and lacks meaning. Depression affects all aspects of life, including:

» Thoughts

» Behaviors

» Feelings

» Relationships

Many people suffer from depression from time to time. They may have a temporary feeling of sadness and pessimism; these feelings are often related to real-life stressors that seem over-whelming. However, when those feelings last longer than a few weeks, the normal feeling of depression becomes a disorder that requires treatment.

What Is Major Depressive Disorder?

Major depressive disorder occurs when sadness, loss of interest, and loss of pleasure persist over weeks. Along with that low mood, other symptoms occur, including:

» *Apathy* (lack of interest or caring)

» Changes in activity level

» Changes in appetite

» Changes in sleep patterns

» Fatigue

» Intense feelings of guilt

>> Loss of self-esteem

>> Poor concentration

>> Thoughts of suicide or death

Someone with major depression may literally have trouble getting out of bed. Dark despair grabs hold of a person's life and squeezes out the possibility of pleasure.

How Does Depression Differ from Sadness or Grief?

When you lose someone or something you love, you experience grief, which includes sadness, fatigue, problems sleeping, changes in appetite, and not being able to get anything done. You may even have thoughts of ending your life.

Like depression, grief ebbs and flows. Unlike depression, grief usually subsides over time. That time varies greatly — months or years. But over time, the pain of grief is not as overwhelming and intense. However, grief that does not resolve can evolve into depression. At that point, professional help is recommended.

TIP

You may be concerned about yourself or someone you care about during the experience of grief. Support groups can be a good source of help. If support groups aren't enough, ask your primary care provider to evaluate whether other treatment is warranted. Or make an appointment with a mental health provider who specializes in grief.

How Common Is Depression?

More than 15 percent of the U.S. population will experience depression during their lifetime. At any one time, about 6 percent to 8 percent of the U.S. population is currently experiencing depression. Young adults and females are more likely to have depression than adult males. Generally, having one major depressive episode puts you at greater risk for relapses, especially without treatment.

Can Depression Be Prevented?

Depression cannot be prevented, but it can be reduced, and the symptoms can be milder with the right interventions. Depression is often connected to stressful events, which can lead to changes in thinking. These patterns of negative thinking include thoughts like the following:

» Everything I do turns out to be wrong.

» Nothing will ever get better for me.

» The world is going to end soon.

When you have insight into your negative thinking patterns, you can catch depression in its early stages and get treatment (see Chapters 9 and 10).

What Are the Different Types of Depression?

Mental health professionals create labels to describe the clusters of symptoms that form types of depression. Although the various forms of depression have similarities, such as sadness and lack of interest, they do have differences. The following are types of depression:

» **Major depressive disorder:** Persistent sadness; lack of interest; changes in appetite and sleep; and feelings of guilt and worthlessness. Sometimes includes a wish to harm oneself.

» **Persistent depressive disorder:** Chronic symptoms of major depression that are milder but last for at least two years.

» **Disruptive mood dysregulation disorder:** Diagnosed in children and adolescents. Chronic irritability and angry outbursts, almost always starting before the age of ten.

» **Premenstrual dysphoric disorder:** Depression, anxiety, and irritability that start prior to a menstrual period and ends shortly after.

» **Seasonal affective disorder:** Symptoms of a major depressive disorder that generally start when the days get shorter in the fall and resolve in the spring.

» **Postpartum depression:** Major depressive symptoms that begin shortly after giving birth.

» **Adjustment disorder with depressed mood:** Depression following a significant loss or trauma that lasts long enough to interfere with daily life.

» **Depression associated with disease or drugs:** Depression caused by or as a result of experiencing a medical condition or as a side effect of a medication or drug.

What's the Difference between Major Depression and Persistent Depressive Disorder?

Think about the difference between a cold and the flu. A cold can be very distressing and annoying, especially if it lingers and persists with a runny nose and a chronic cough. However, when necessary, most people with colds can muddle through the day. They're able to get dressed, feed themselves, and do what needs to be done. They may feel tired and may take a nap.

Now consider the flu. The fever, nausea, and aches and pains of the flu often make it impossible to get the smallest thing done. Many people with the flu need to stay in bed and, at most, eat some crackers or toast.

Persistent depressive disorder (formerly known as *dysthymia*) is more like a cold — lots of people with persistent depressive disorder function, just not as well. Major depression, on the other hand, is like the flu — those with major depression have a difficult time getting through the day.

TIP

Throughout this book, I use the term *depression* to describe the various symptoms that are usually associated with major depressive disorder.

What's the Difference between Depression and Bipolar Disorder?

Depression and bipolar disorder have some similarities, but they aren't the same. Both conditions generally involve a depressed mood for periods of time. And when a person is depressed, symptoms include sadness, sleep problems, eating changes, and loss of pleasure.

However, in bipolar disorder, moods swing — sometimes from deep depression to extreme mania. Manic symptoms include restless energy, sleeplessness, risky behaviors, poor decision-making, talking too fast, and extremely poor judgment.

What's the Difference between Depression and Anxiety?

Anxiety and depression are the two most common mental health disorders. They can both be highly disruptive and interfere with normal functioning. Both can result in poor sleep, change in appetite, and a tendency to isolate. However, they have distinct symptoms.

Depression involves sadness, pessimism, loss of pleasure, and fatigue. Anxiety is a fear-based reaction; it's accompanied by significant physical symptoms such as elevated heart rate, sweaty hands, stomach upset, and muscle aches. Untreated, anxiety can lead to depression.

DID YOU KNOW?

Many people believe that depression results from a chemical imbalance in the brain. Despite decades of research, scientists still really don't know exactly how that works or what causes it. What we do know is that many people benefit from medications that change brain chemistry.

Chapter **2**

The Biology of Depression

The brain and biology play a big role in depression. The various systems are inter-related, and science continues to find more connections. This chapter answers basic questions about the structure and function of the brain, brain chemicals, and the digestive system — and their reciprocal relationship to depression.

How Does Depression Affect the Brain?

Depression is associated with emotions such as hopelessness, sadness, lack of joy, and apathy. Depression also affects the brain. These changes are extremely unique in each individual and may not occur in every brain. The following changes are common:

» Reduced volume in certain brain regions, which can impact emotional responses, memory, and thinking ability

» Differences in the levels of neurotransmitters, which can affect sleep, mood, appetite, and drive

» Increased levels of stress hormones

» Increased activity in areas of the brain that regulate emotional responses

What's fascinating about these brain changes is that the brain returns to normal when treatment is successful. And treatment can be psychotherapy or medication (or both).

What Is the Role of Neurotransmitters in Depression?

The brain has about 100 billion *neurons* (cells that receive information from the outside world and direct responses in the body). Neurons communicate by way of chemical messengers called *neurotransmitters.* Depression occurs when the chemical conversations between neurons break down.

Three major neurotransmitters are related to depression:

» **Serotonin:** Regulates mood, sleep, and appetite

» **Norepinephrine:** Related to problems with energy, decreased attention, and fatigue

» **Dopamine:** Has to do with pleasure, motivation, and alertness

Is Depression Caused by a Chemical Imbalance?

The chemical imbalance theory of depression has been debunked. Depression has many causes (see Chapter 3), but despite advertising champaigns to convince people to ask their doctors for medication to balance their chemicals, no evidence to date has confirmed that depression is caused by having too much or too little of a certain chemical. For example, if lack of serotonin were the cause of depression, an IV of serotonin would likely work — but it doesn't.

That doesn't mean that brain chemistry plays no part in depression — it does. But it's the age-old question: Which comes first? In this case, it's likely that other causes come first and that brain imbalances are the result of such things as trauma, hormonal changes, chronic stress, or genetic influences.

How Does the Brain's Structure and Function Relate to Depression?

The brain structure of some people with depression shows loss of brain volume including in the area that processes emotions (called the *amygdala*) and the area that is responsible for memory and stress reactivity (the *hippocampus*). These changes appear to be temporary and improve with treatment.

The function of the brain is also impacted by depression. Higher-level decision-making such as planning, largely controlled by the prefrontal cortex, appears underactive. The emotional processing center is overactive. Therefore, a depressed person can easily make decisions that aren't carefully thought out based on emotions that are overactive.

How Does the Gut–Brain Connection Affect Depression?

Recently more attention has been paid to the relationship between the brain and the digestive system. The gut–brain connection is bidirectional. For example, you have a life filled with chronic stress, which is often a precursor to depression; stress leads to bouts of diarrhea, loss of appetite, constipation, or nausea, and those symptoms can lead to inflammation, changes in neurotransmitters, and low mood.

Similarly, you can have chronic gastrointestinal symptoms such as gastroesophageal reflux disease (GERD), irritable bowel syndrome (IBS), peptic ulcer, or inflammatory bowel disease (IBD), which can lead to anxiety and depression. The gut–brain connection can be a well-working team or a vicious cycle.

DID YOU KNOW?

Many people with depression hide it very well. On the outside, they appear fine, happy even. However, deep inside, they're suffering. Although they push through the day, they can hardly get out the door. They listlessly drink a cup of coffee and down a protein shake. But when they arrive at work, they put on a happy face. No one knows how miserable they are inside. That's one reason depression is often called an invisible disease.

Chapter **3**

The Root Causes of Depression

This chapter examines many factors that can lead to depression. Usually, there's more than one reason that someone gets depressed. Often, multiple factors interact with each other.

For instance, if someone is prone to depression because of genetic history and then they lose their home due to a forest fire, they may experience depression. However, their next-door neighbor, who also lost their home, but doesn't have a genetic predisposition, is able to gather themselves together and move on through the difficult process of rebuilding.

In this chapter, I take a look at the various causes associated with the development of depression.

What Causes Depression?

Depression can be caused by biological, social, or psychological factors. For example, some depression may largely be caused by trauma. Another person's depression may be a complication of grief. A third person was born with a genetic predisposition for depression. Someone else may be lonely. And most people with depression have a combination of factors that lead to their despair.

How Do Life Events and Trauma Contribute to Depression?

When people experience trauma, they may also feel helpless. Traumatic events often happen unexpectedly and are usually unpreventable. For example, a child who is abused did not choose to be abused, nor did a crime victim ask to be victimized. Similarly, someone who experienced a traumatic event such as a natural disaster or a war does not choose to be in the wrong place at the wrong time. Following traumatic events, if the person feels hopeless, is pessimistic about the future, and loses self-esteem, depression is likely to occur.

Most people have an immediate reaction to trauma and then recover. Others can become chronically depressed. Multiple factors — such as childhood experiences, physical health, previous mental health issues, and resilience — determine individual reactions to trauma.

In addition to trauma, life events such as an impoverished or difficult childhood, poor educational opportunities, discrimination, job-related problems, or social isolation all contribute to the chances of developing depression.

Can Medical Conditions Cause Depression?

Medical conditions can cause depression in three different ways:

>> **People may become depressed that they have a certain medical condition.** Who wouldn't be depressed about having cancer, heart disease, or a chronic disease such as diabetes?

» **Being sick interferes with everyday life such as work, getting together with friends, and having enjoyable meals.** This can lead to depression.

» **Medical conditions can also affect the nervous system in ways that create depression.** Diseases such as cancer, asthma, coronary artery disease, multiple sclerosis, Parkinson's disease, thyroid disease, and stroke in particular are thought to contribute to depression. As in many relationships, the question "Which comes first?" is impossible to answer.

Can Depression Be a Side Effect of Other Mental Health Conditions?

Anxiety disorders, especially untreated, often lead to depression. Other disorders common with depression include substance abuse, eating disorders, or personality disorders.

The unrelenting disturbance of other mental health conditions frequently leads to serious depression. The stress of living with these conditions can trigger a depressive reaction. People with a history of trauma or abuse may be more vulnerable than others.

How Do Hormonal Changes Affect Depression?

Hormones interact with chemicals in the brain and affect mood. Some changes increase depressive symptoms. Often thought of as primarily a problem with women, men can also have mood swings when the male hormone testosterone changes.

The following hormones are thought to be most involved in mood regulation:

» **Estrogen:** The female hormone that fluctuates during menstruation, postpartum, and menopause is linked to an increase in depressive symptoms.

» **Progesterone:** Fluctuations may increase irritability or moodiness.

» **Testosterone:** Low levels in men may increase risk of depression and moodiness.

» **Thyroid hormones:** Too much or too little is linked to irritability, moodiness, and depression.

What Is the Relationship between Depression and Substance Abuse?

Depressed people frequently turn to alcohol or drugs in an attempt to quell the pain and distress of the disease. Unfortunately, they may inadvertently increase their depression in the long run. Chronic substance abuse can also lead to depression. Like many of these relationships, depression and substance abuse become a vicious cycle, feeding off each other.

How Does Chronic Stress Impact Depression?

Chronic stress can be a risk factor for depression. However, depression is not an inevitable result of chronic stress. Some people are able to withstand chronic stress; others thrive on it. When people believe that chronic stress is unrelenting, that they do not have any control over the situation, and that the future is bleak, they may become depressed.

Can Depression Be Triggered by Certain Medications?

Some medications do directly cause depressive symptoms. It's difficult to determine how much the medication is contributing versus how much the illness is contributing to symptoms. However, medications such as anticonvulsants for seizures, benzodiazepines for anxiety, high blood pressure medications, hormones, steroids, levodopa for Parkinson's, statins for high cholesterol, and some drugs to treat cancer can cause depressed mood. Many other drugs may have similar effects.

Usually, when conditions improve, or after a few weeks, side effects are minimal. However, if depression lingers, talk with your medical provider.

TIP

How Do Environmental Factors Influence Depression?

Studies show that environmental stress such as air pollution, overcrowding, noise, and toxins can lead to anxiety or depression. Toxins in the environment cause changes in the brain of those exposed. Long-term exposure is more likely to lead to problems than short-term exposure.

As with other triggers, more than one factor is almost always at work. For example, people living in poverty are generally more likely to also live in an area with high rates of environmental toxins, noxious noise levels, and overcrowding. It's impossible to quantify the relative potency of each individual risk factor.

What Is Seasonal Affective Disorder?

Seasonal affective disorder (SAD) is a major depressive disorder that is associated with changes in the amount of light in the day. Those with SAD usually experience low mood during the late fall and winter months. Symptoms that appear to be common and somewhat unique to SAD include the need for more sleep and increased appetite. Some experts speculate that, like bears preparing to hibernate for the winter, people are establishing a cozy cave with full bellies, ready for the winter season.

Can Poor Diet and Nutrition Contribute to Depression?

We have a lot to learn about the brain–gut connection, but research does show a relationship between poor diet and increased depression. Highly processed foods — such as potato chips, sugar-filled sodas, cookies, and processed meats — contribute to inflammation, which appears to increase depression risk.

Those whose diet is rich in whole foods such as fruits, vegetables, unprocessed grains, and olive oil have a lower risk of depression.

Again, interactions between many variables make determining the actual amount of risk impossible. More definitive data about these complex relationships will likely emerge in the future.

How Does Sleep Deprivation Impact Depression?

Not getting enough sleep for a night or two isn't a big deal. And some people can get by perfectly fine on a few hours of good sleep a night. For most people, chronic sleep deprivation leads to depressed mood. Interestingly, depression often leads to insomnia, so like almost all the factors mentioned in this chapter, there is an bidirectional interaction between depression and sleep deprivation.

DID YOU KNOW?

Interesting research over the years has supported a theory called the disability paradox, *which happens when people rank their happiness before and after a spinal cord injury. Interestingly, their levels of happiness remain basically the same. For example, someone who reported that they were usually happy before an accident recovered their level of happiness even after experiencing a disability such as paralysis and reliance on a wheelchair. After a brief period of shock and rehabilitation, people are amazingly resilient.*

Chapter **4**

Other Risk Factors

The causes of depression are multiple. In this chapter, I look at social and cultural factors as possible contributors to depression. New devices, old prejudices, economic challenges, or cultural differences all impact functioning and levels of stress. That stress can lead to depression in some people but not in others. This chapter explains why.

How Does Social Media Impact Rates of Depression?

Studies show that the rate of depression has gone up in tandem with the use of smartphones. Depression, especially among teenagers, young adults, and women, continues to increase as more time is spent on social media. Research indicates that long hours spent scrolling on social media lead to a greater incidence of poor mental health in general, including depression.

Scrolling increases social isolation, a risk factor for depression. In addition, the act of *social comparison* (comparing your life to others) contributes to low self-esteem. It's difficult to measure up to the artificial standards of social media.

How Does Bullying Increase Rates of Depression?

Incivility can lead to depression. When someone experiences incivility, they feel socially rejected and criticized. In addition, the chronic nature of incivility, either at home or in the workplace, wears down resilience, leading to emotional exhaustion.

The ultimate act of incivility is bullying. Bullying occurs when one person perceives themselves as having more power — whether physical, social, or financial — and uses that power to belittle, taunt, or control someone else. Sometimes the bully uses embarrassing information about their victim to get them to do what they want.

Being bullied hurts self-esteem. It leads to feelings of powerlessness, hopelessness, and helplessness, all risk factors for depression. Cyberbullying can induce a trauma response in its victims, depending on the severity. Victims often experience lasting negative effects on their mental health.

Do Political Divisions Increase Depression?

Political divisions sometimes lead families to disengage, friendships to suffer, and broader social networks to collapse. The resulting isolation indeed raises the risk of depression.

In addition, the intensity of political polarization along with a constant barrage of news feeds contribute to feelings of pessimism and hopelessness. The chronic stress of negative commentary and dire predictions for the future lead to emotional exhaustion. Those who follow politics are apparently more likely to experience depressive symptoms associated with political polarization than those who do not follow such news.

Does Discrimination Impact Depression?

People suffer from discrimination based on race, gender, sexual identity, class, social status, ethnicity, and political persuasion. Like other life stressors, unrelenting chronic experiences of discrimination lead to poor mental health outcomes, including depression.

Discrimination can be subtle or blatant. It contaminates communities and families. When a child is discriminated against, the parents often feel angry and hopeless. When hate crimes are committed, whole communities may mourn.

TIP

Chronic stress is a causal factor for depression. The chronic nature of discrimination increases rates of depression in vulnerable populations.

Does Financial Hardship Increase Depression?

Financial insecurity and instability lead to higher rates of depression in those who are affected. Economic inequality is at its greatest, and the erosion of the middle class has been documented. Families are burdened by student loans and unaffordable housing. There is great uncertainty about how artificial intelligence (AI) will disrupt the workforce and the jobs of the future. No wonder stress levels are high.

Many people consider money and wealth integral parts of their own self-worth. When people can't meet their obligations, they may experience great guilt and lower self-esteem. These factors, along with chronic stress, increase rates of depression.

Is Depression More Common in Certain Cultures?

Across the world, all people suffer from sadness, grief, and loss. However, some cultures do not recognize those feelings as symptoms of a mental illness. They view the withdrawal and loss of interest as natural feelings in response to a life event. In fact, in some languages there is no translation of the word *depression.*

Accordingly, it's often thought that depression is more prevalent in modern, Western culture. That's hard to quantify because of differences in expression and describing symptoms. For example, in Japan, mental illness is more likely to be thought of as unacceptable, so most people with symptoms won't admit them openly. Does that mean that Japan's rate of depression is lower than that of other countries? Not necessarily. It just may be more hidden.

What research does suggest is that focus on the individual, on the self, may be linked to more depression. This individualistic culture stresses independence and autonomy. In cultures that stress cooperation and collectivism, more satisfaction may be derived from group membership and support available when life is challenging.

2

The Symptoms and Side Effects of Depression

This part walks through the symptoms of depression, including its impacts on the body and behavior. It also explains the impact of depression on relationships and social interactions.

DID YOU KNOW?

Depression is a disease of extremes — from ravenous hunger to feeling sick at the sight of food, from insomnia to sleeping all day and night, from frantic pacing to collapse.

Chapter **5**

Symptoms of Depression

Each case of depression is unique. There is no specific checklist that must be satisfied to get a diagnosis of depression. However, clusters of symptoms are generally consistent with the diagnosis. These symptoms involve thoughts, emotions, and physical sensations. This chapter spells out the symptoms usually associated with the disorder.

What Are the Early Signs of Depression?

Early signs of depression are mild symptoms of depression. You may feel a lack of enjoyment of previously fun experiences, but not much sadness. Or you may not feel like getting together with friends but still attend family functions when necessary.

Early depression may involve poor appetite or a desire to eat lots of chips. It may involve having a hard time getting things done and procrastinating. These signs may not be evident to the person or the outside world, but they are warnings that storms may be on the horizon.

What Are the Emotional Symptoms of Depression?

The major emotion of depression is persistent sadness and misery. A person with depression may also feel helpless, which turns into hopelessness about the future. In addition, there is a loss of interest in work, people, or activities that were once meaningful or pleasurable. Someone with depression is also likely to lack patience and feel easily irritated.

Self-loathing and guilt round out the emotional symptoms of depression. Those two emotions may lead to the desire to "check out," or disappear from life. In other words, low self-worth and misery, combined with hopelessness, may increase the risk of self-harming behaviors or suicide.

What Are the Physical Symptoms of Depression?

Most people diagnosed with depression also feel sluggish, run down, and tired. Fatigue is a major physical symptom of depression. That fatigue may cause them to sleep too much. On the other hand, some people with depression suffer from insomnia — they're either not able to fall asleep or unable to go back to sleep after waking in the early hours, or both.

Appetite changes are also common with depression. Some people have no appetite and can barely force themselves to eat. Others can't seem to get enough and are rarely satiated.

Muscle aches and pains, headaches, and stomach upsets are also typical physical symptoms of depression. This chronic discomfort has no known physical cause; these feelings are simply ones of general malaise.

What Are the Cognitive Symptoms of Depression?

Depression affects thinking abilities. People who are depressed have sluggish thinking. They may feel like they can't keep up with conversations, lack concentration, and drift in and out of social interactions. They may feel confused and at times untypically forgetful. Slowed speech and thinking complete the picture of suffering.

Can Depression Symptoms Change over Time?

Depression can be classified as mild, moderate, or severe. These descriptions rate the frequency, intensity, and duration of symptoms. Those with mild depression may be able to function, just at a reduced level. However, those with severe depression are often unable to work and complete their daily responsibilities.

These changes in severity can be related to

» Successful or unsuccessful treatment
» Differing environments that either increase or reduce stress
» Unknown reasons

DID YOU KNOW?

When a professional athlete suffers an injury, they're very likely to become depressed. That's because their personal identity is wrapped up in their performance. The lack of purpose and loss of self-worth can lead to feelings of uselessness and hopelessness. Unfortunately, depression can slow the healing process, so a vicious cycle is formed.

Chapter **6**

Physical and Behavioral Impacts of Depression

Depression is an illness of the mind and the body. In this chapter, I explore various physical symptoms of depression.

How Does Depression Affect Sleep?

Depression disrupts the natural sleep–wake cycle known as the *circadian rhythm.* Therefore, normal sleep patterns can be disturbed. People with depression may find that they're sleepy during the day and wide awake at night.

Depression also changes the hormones and neurotransmitters in the brain. There may be imbalances in the brain chemicals that regulate sleep, as well as increased levels of stress hormones that keep people awake.

In addition, negative thinking, *ruminating* (having repetitive, intrusive thoughts), and worrying interfere with sleep. Especially during early morning awakening, the depressed mind can form an endless loop of negative thinking.

Can Depression Cause Changes in Appetite or Weight?

The relationship between depression, appetite, and changes in weight is complicated. One area of the brain that depression affects is the reward system. People with depression report a loss of pleasure. When that extends to eating, some people lose their appetite and lose weight.

Depression is twice as likely to occur in people who are obese. Although some people may lose the desire to eat, others may engage in emotional eating. Emotional eating often includes foods high in fat, sugar, or carbohydrates.

A cognitive symptom of depression, *apathy* (lack of interest or caring), may also make committing to a healthy lifestyle more challenging. In addition, antidepressants can lead to nausea and weight loss or, more commonly, weight gain. The bottom line is that depression leads to changes in appetite, changes in eating habits, and changes in weight.

How Does Depression Affect Attention and Focus?

Depression makes it difficult to sustain focus on important tasks and ignore distractions. This ability, called *selective attention,* is crucial to getting through the day safely. Important tasks range from the mundane (like getting gas in the tank) to critical (like not driving while distracted). Running out of gas is not as dangerous as running into another car. Distraction can be deadly.

Depression also interferes with the ability to sustain attention or maintain focus on a certain task, such as school or work. Finally, depression negatively impacts the ability to switch attention between tasks, commonly known as *multitasking.*

How Does Depression Influence Decision-Making?

Decision-making is a complex mental task. It involves attention, memory, problem-solving, and considering future implications. Depression causes lack of focus and fatigue, which lead to indecisiveness and decreased ability to gather the resources to make informed decisions.

Furthermore, depression leads to a negative bias. Those who are depressed tend to see the world through dark glasses. They're likely to be pessimistic and predict negative outcomes, which makes decision-making difficult and likely inaccurate.

Can Depression Cause Memory Problems?

Depression affects brain function. It may cause inflammation, which can lead to memory impairment. Some people with depression show shrinkage in the *hippocampus,* a part of the brain that supports memory. In addition, neurochemicals that are crucial to memory are disrupted with depression. Finally, stress interferes with memory.

The types of memory impaired during depressive episodes include:

- » **Short-term memory:** Forgetting the name of someone you just met or why you walked into a room
- » **Working memory:** Making decisions, holding multiple items in memory at once, following a recipe, or figuring out a schedule
- » **Long-term memory:** Memories of past experiences or personal details; usually less impaired by depressive episodes
- » **Memory retrieval:** Forgetting words or names that you usually recall

Can Depression Cause Physical Pain?

Depression and pain form a vicious cycle. More pain, more depression. More depression, more pain. Pain is likely related to disruptions in the neurotransmitter system in the brain and chronic inflammation that goes along with depression. Common symptoms include:

- » Headaches
- » Muscle and joint aches
- » Back pain
- » Neck pain
- » Stomach upset
- » Fatigue

How Does Depression Impact Motivation and Energy Levels?

Many people with depression express a feeling of overwhelming fatigue. They feel like they're walking in mud, struggling to slog through, but find themselves almost entirely at a standstill. In addition to fatigue, a great sense of apathy reigns. Nothing seems important enough to get done. Not only that, but pleasure is almost erased from their lives, giving them little incentive to accomplish much.

Unfortunately, everyday responsibilities are often not completed, and those failures add to their sense of hopelessness and helplessness. Depression deepens, as does their poor sense of self-worth.

Can Depression Cause Irritability or Anger?

Emotional regulation is the ability to acknowledge emotions and express them in a way that's appropriate to the setting and situation. For example, if you were at a PTA meeting, you probably wouldn't tell your child's teacher that their breath stinks even though you're feeling disgusted by it. At best, you might offer the teacher a mint.

When people are depressed, their ability to regulate their own emotions is decreased. Their ability to handle frustration is also decreased, which results in irritability and sometimes angry outbursts. This pattern is more common among depressed adolescents and men.

Can Depression Cause Suicidal Thoughts?

Most people with mild depression do not have suicidal thoughts. They feel down and sad, not even close to wanting to end their lives. However, for those suffering from moderate to severe depression, suicidal thoughts, also called *ideation,* are more common.

When depression is accompanied by helplessness and hopelessness, the risk is greater. Furthermore, when substance abuse is present, when there has been a previous suicide attempt, when there is a family history of suicide, and when the person has access to deadly means, the risk is greater.

If you have suicidal thoughts, call or text 988. If danger to self or others is imminent, dial 911 and report a mental health emergency.

DID YOU KNOW?

The cost of depression to the U.S. economy is almost $300 billion a year. That's about the same amount of money that a recession would likely cost. Most of the cost is because of lost wages, unemployment, and increased healthcare costs.

Chapter **7**

Relationships and Social Impact

Depression changes the way people relate to each other. When a person feels depressed, they turn away from the very people who would support them. They withdraw and avoid others. Sometimes people with depression become critical and irritable with those around them. Friends then also avoid those with depression because they're uncomfortable being around someone so crabby and down. No wonder depression leads to more loneliness and isolation.

How Does Depression Affect Daily Life?

Depression slows down life. All aspects of life are impacted by depression. It's hard to get out of bed, eat properly, accomplish tasks, and sleep comfortably. Depression snuffs out optimism and quashes curiosity. Listless attention causes errors, and loss of interest makes work seem impossible.

How Does Depression Impact Intimate Relationships?

Partners and family members of people with depression often feel dismissed. Depression causes people to become self-centered. They dwell on how miserable they are, neglecting the people in their lives. They lack the energy to be good parents, partners, or friends.

After repeatedly trying to connect, the friends and family of those with depression become frustrated. This leads to hurt feelings and sometimes withdrawal. When intimate partners withdraw, the depressed person may feel rejected and withdraw further.

How Does Depression Affect Social Interactions?

When people are depressed, they don't want to interact with others. Period. No amount of social life can lift someone out of depression. Interacting with others is a chore, not something to be desired.

When interactions are necessary, someone with depression may seem disinterested, distracted, and even irritated. Other people may believe that the person with depression is uptight, angry, or snobbish. In reality, the person is probably suffering silently, unable to make themselves be socially engaged.

Can Lack of Social Support Contribute to Depression?

Not having social support is a risk factor for depression. Loneliness and isolation increase the likelihood of depression and even suicide. Those who lack people in their lives believe that there is no one to turn to. They don't ask for help, even when others are quite willing to intervene.

People with poor relationships are also at greater risk for depression. Those who have disruptive, confrontational, and particularly violent relationships do not enjoy the protective factor of positive social relationships.

In addition, loss of important relationships can slightly increase the risk of depression. Most people experience grief after a loss, which gradually decreases over time. Those whose grief does not decrease with time may develop depression. People who lose relationships after a period of intense conflict are also at greater risk for depression.

Does Poor Physical Health Cause Depression?

Chronic illness, especially when pain is not controlled, is certainly a risk factor for depression. Studies suggest that between 25 percent and 50 percent of those who suffer from chronic conditions have depression.

Illnesses such as heart disease and diabetes, as well as chronic pain conditions, lead to changes in lifestyle. These changes usually involve a restriction of pleasurable activities and sometimes social isolation.

Like many other factors that increase the risk, a vicious cycle is at work. When someone is depressed, pain increases, and the illness often gets worse. And the worsening symptoms lead to more depression.

How Does Depression Affect Self-Esteem?

Unlike the optimistic outlook of those wearing rose-colored glasses, those with depression wear very dark glasses that produce a pessimistic scene. They see the worst possible present, predict the direst future, and look back at a past pockmarked by failure.

This focus on failure leads to feelings of worthlessness and poor self-esteem. When something good happens or something positive is accomplished, the person with depression is likely to attribute it to good luck instead of acknowledging something encouraging.

Can Depression Cause Feelings of Guilt or Worthlessness?

Those same dark-colored glasses don't allow a depressed person to see that others may care about them or that their lives have any value. Low self-esteem and worthlessness go together. Worthless people believe that they're incapable of being productive or having positive relationships. So, feeling worthless and inept, depressed people tend to isolate themselves, which exacerbates their depression.

In addition, looking back, those with depression tend to blame themselves for failure even if they weren't responsible. They feel sad that they aren't the best partner, friend, parent, or colleague because of their depression. And they see a future of not being good enough. Thus, guilt becomes a frequent companion.

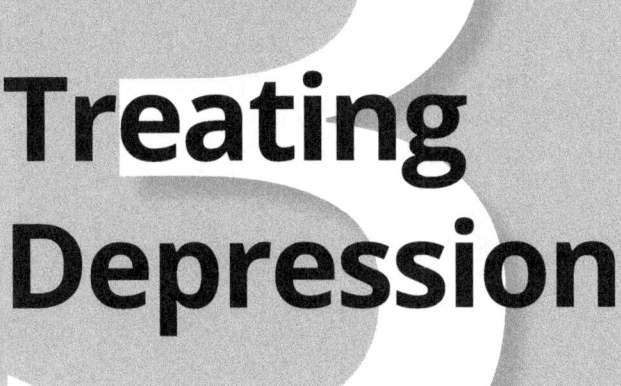

3

Treating
Depression

IN THIS PART . . .

This part explains how depression is diagnosed by a medical professional and how it's treated. It also walks you through the various therapeutic approaches to depression, from cognitive behavioral therapy to interpersonal therapy and more.

DID YOU KNOW?

With treatment, between 80 percent and 90 percent of people with depression find symptom relief. That's great news. The first step toward successful treatment is getting an accurate diagnosis.

Chapter **8**

Diagnosing Depression

When someone has a cluster of symptoms that are interfering with their ability to participate fully in their life, they may have depression. Depression is a serious mental health condition that can be controlled with effective treatment. With a correct diagnosis and treatment plan, the prognosis is good. This chapter answers questions about how to get there.

How Is Depression Diagnosed?

Depression is diagnosed by a healthcare provider when a person presents with a number of symptoms such as sadness, lack of pleasure, changes in eating or sleeping habits, low self-esteem, and feelings of worthlessness. These symptoms must have persisted for at least a couple of weeks. After an interview including history of symptoms, severity of symptoms, and persistence of symptoms, a diagnosis is given.

Depression should be diagnosed by a trained licensed mental health provider. However, most depression is diagnosed by primary care providers. Most of the time, that works out — the primary care provider often starts treatment with an antidepressant. Unfortunately, sometimes depression is not the correct diagnosis and treatment with medication doesn't work.

TIP

A trained psychologist, psychiatrist, or other mental health professional is best equipped to rule out other causes of the symptoms of depression. For example, grief is not considered depression, although it sometimes turns into depression. And some people with mood disorders present to their primary care provider with symptoms of depression but need different care because of their unique underlying needs.

Can Depression Be Misdiagnosed?

Physical illness often mimics depression. For example, extreme fatigue can be a symptom of depression, hormonal imbalances, or anemia. Forgetfulness is found both in depression and dementia. Irritability happens with diabetes. Changes in sleeping or eating habits occur with anxiety disorders, medication side effects, or depression. And low mood can happen in people with bipolar disorder as well as depression.

TIP

A thorough and accurate diagnosis is imperative so that treatment is appropriate. A delay in care because of misdiagnosis leads to poor quality of life.

What's the PHQ-9 Assessment?

The Patient Health Questionnaire-9 (PHQ-9) is a free screening test used for diagnosing and measuring the symptoms and severity of depression. Nine symptoms are listed:

» Depressed mood
» Loss of interest or pleasure
» Sleep disturbances
» Changes in appetite
» Unexplained fatigue

- » Problems concentrating
- » Moving or speaking slowly or fidgeting or chattering more than usual
- » Feeling guilty or worthless
- » Thoughts of self-harm or suicide

You read each statement and rate whether you have the symptoms on a 0 (not at all) to 3 (almost every day) scale. The ratings are added together, with a total ranging from 0 to 27. The higher the score, the higher the severity of depression.

The PHQ-9 is often used as a stand-alone evaluation. However, a professional should also conduct a diagnostic interview to further clarify the possible diagnosis.

When Should I Seek Professional Help for Depression?

If symptoms of depression last more than a few weeks, if your everyday life is negatively impacted, and if your relationships are strained, you should be evaluated. That's because treatment can be very effective. Start with your primary care provider to quickly rule out other possible physical causes such as a reaction to a medication or a hormone imbalance. They may also be able to provide you with a referral to a mental health professional.

How Do I Find the Right Therapist for My Depression?

Some people spend more time picking out the best avocado at the grocery store than they do choosing a therapist. Taking the time necessary to find a good match is well worth it. Getting a good therapist can help you recover from depression. Finding a bad fit will lead to wasted time and possibly increased emotional distress. When you're considering a therapist, pay attention to the following:

» **Training and licensure:** Make sure that your therapist is licensed by your state and trained in an empirically supported therapy (see Chapter 10 for more information about types of therapy for depression).

» **Reputation and recommendations:** Ask your primary care provider for a referral. Ask trusted friends or family members who have been in therapy for recommendations. Check the state licensing board for any complaints. Therapists can't ask for public recommendations because of privacy concerns.

» **Financial:** Check with your insurance company to see if it covers psychotherapy. Most insurance plans do, however it may have a restricted number of visits or have a panel of its own providers. If you're paying out of pocket, be sure to ask about fees and possible sliding scales.

» **Scheduling:** Many mental health providers have extremely full practices. Make sure that you can come up with some potential times that work for both of you. Virtual visits make scheduling easier for many clients and providers.

What Should I Expect during My First Appointment for Depression?

During the first appointment with a mental health professional, you'll likely go over confidentiality. Therapy is sort of like going to confession — you can tell your therapist all about your darkest thoughts and secrets and assume that those words will be kept private. Like your doctor or priest, your therapist is bound by law and ethics to keep your private information confidential.

There are a couple of exceptions to confidentiality: If you tell your therapist that you're about to kill yourself or seriously harm someone else, the therapist is legally required to get the help necessary to keep you and others safe. Additionally, if you're abusing a child or an elder, those behaviors also have to be reported.

In addition to confidentiality, your therapist will ask lots of questions about your mental health history, your symptoms, and their severity.

What Questions Should I Ask My Therapist about Depression?

Ask your therapist about their experience working with people who have depression. In addition, ask them whether they use empirically validated approaches to treat depression.

Also, ask your therapist how long therapy typically takes, what the immediate goals of therapy are, and what techniques they'll be using.

What Should I Do If I Feel My Treatment Isn't Working?

Sometimes therapy doesn't work. It could be that your therapist looks just like your last boyfriend who dumped you or you can't stand the way your therapist coughs. If that's the case, take the time to talk to your therapist about your concerns. You may be able to resolve some minor issues.

However, if you don't feel comfortable talking to your therapist, or if you feel like your therapist isn't listening to you, you probably have a bigger problem going on. If you don't feel that treatment is working, talk to your therapist about your worries.

If talking doesn't help or if you feel judged, change therapists — especially if you don't feel safe.

TIP

Don't judge your therapist for at least a couple of weeks, unless your concerns are very significant. It often takes a bit of time to feel comfortable with a new therapist, so try not to jump ship before you give yourself and your therapist a chance.

How Can I Advocate for Myself in the Healthcare System?

Being an advocate for yourself in the healthcare system leads to better care and better outcomes. First, educate yourself about your rights to care. Check out your insurance and find out what it pays and what it doesn't. How does your insurance handle referrals?

Armed with that information, find out as much as you can about your mental or physical health conditions. If you have depression, look at information from reliable sources (such as Mayo Clinic, WebMD, or the Centers for Disease Control and Prevention), about treatment options. Also take time to learn about symptoms, severity, duration, and complications of the condition.

TIP

When you get healthcare, feel free to take notes during the session. Some providers will even allow you to record sessions. Discuss your treatment and goals with your provider.

DID YOU KNOW?

One of the symptoms of depression is loss of pleasure, which may result in a loss of appetite. However, weight loss is not as common as weight gain in depression. That may be because people lose interest in eating a healthy diet and exercising.

Chapter **9**

Treatment Options

D epression, a common mental health condition, is highly treatable. This chapter examines treatments for depression and their outcomes.

What Are the Treatment Options for Depression?

The two most common treatment options for depression are psychotherapy and medication. Therapy and medication are often combined. In addition, lifestyle modifications and certain brain stimulations are often supplemental or given when psychotherapy and medication are ineffective.

How Effective Is Therapy for Depression?

Psychotherapy is very effective for depression. In fact, many people find that psychotherapy alone helps alleviate symptoms to the point of complete remission. Therapy helps people solve problems, take different perspectives, and decrease negative thinking. The success of therapy depends on a well-trained skilled therapist, a good relationship between client and therapist, and a client willing to implement techniques learned in therapy in real life.

TIP

In addition to working well to decrease symptoms, psychotherapy doesn't come with the side effects of medication, and it appears to be better at preventing relapse.

Can Medication Help with Depression?

Medication can be an effective treatment for depression. Unfortunately, only about 60 percent of people respond to medication with a significant reduction in symptoms. A similar number of people get better with psychotherapy. And about the same get better with time.

These statistics make medication decisions difficult. Some people find that the first medication prescribed doesn't work, but another one may. For severe depression, it's important to work closely with a mental health professional.

Medication is usually called for if:

» You have suicidal thoughts.

» You have bipolar disorder or depression with psychosis.

» You've tried therapy and it hasn't worked.

» Your symptoms are primarily physical.

» Medical problems are causing your depression.

» You have other mental health issues at the same time.

» Your insurance doesn't cover therapy.

» Your depression is severe.

What Are the Common Antidepressant Medications?

Antidepressants are classified by how they affect one or more of the neurotransmitters in the brain. Neurotransmitters have different symptoms associated with them:

» **Serotonin:** Insomnia, anxiety, sadness, seasonal affective disorder

» **Dopamine:** Poor attention, apathy, loss of pleasure, loss of motivation

» **Norepinephrine:** Lack of energy, decreased alertness, lethargy

The most common antidepressants are called selective serotonin reuptake inhibitors (SSRIs). These medications are usually the first choice because they have fewer side effects than other antidepressants. SSRIs increase the availability of serotonin in the brain.

Other medications include serotonin/norepinephrine reuptake inhibitors (SNRIs), which increase serotonin and norepinephrine, as well as norepinephrine/dopamine reuptake inhibitors (NDRIs), which boost norepinephrine and dopamine.

Many other antidepressants are available, but these are the most commonly prescribed. Older antidepressants also change the neurotransmitters in the brain, but they usually have more side effects.

How Long Does It Take for Antidepressants to Work?

A few people notice an improvement in mood almost immediately after starting antidepressant medication, but that's rare. For most people, antidepressants take two to eight weeks to start working. If you're not feeling any different after eight weeks, it's time to talk to your provider. Talk to your provider if you experience significant side effects as well.

What Are the Side Effects of Antidepressant Medications?

More than a third of people prescribed antidepressant medication stop taking them because of side effects. Though most side effects go away with time, some don't, and others cause considerable distress. Common side effects include:

» Nausea

» Diarrhea

» Headaches

» Dizziness

» Insomnia

» Dry mouth

» Weight gain

» Apathy

» Sexual dysfunction

It's no wonder that so many people stop taking their meds. But before you stop taking your medication, talk to your provider. Many antidepressants need to be tapered, or side effects can be considerable.

Can Alternative Therapies Be Effective for Depression?

Some people don't want to take medication or seek psychotherapy to treat depression. Others may be looking for more natural treatments or a supplement to the treatment that they're already receiving. Complementary or alternative treatments for depression have some research to support it, but for the most part, randomized controlled studies have not been conducted. Possible treatments include:

» Massage

» Acupuncture

» Vitamins

» Herbs

» Aromatherapy

» Hypnosis

» Meditation

» Yoga

» Chiropractic services

These strategies are probably harmless — and they may help. Talk to your healthcare provider about any supplements that you're considering — they may have interactions with drugs that you're already taking. (See Chapters 12 and 13 for more information about self-management strategies for depression.)

Can Depression Be Cured?

The good news is that with all the available treatments, depression *can* be successfully treated. After treatment, people can lead happy, productive lives. However, the relapse rate for depression is quite high. About half of those who have experienced one major depressive disorder have a relapse. The rate goes up as people have more bouts of depression. Good news again: Relapse can also be successfully treated.

Sadness is a normal human emotion. So, don't expect that getting treatment for depression will keep you from getting sad again. Life is full of challenges and loss. Plus, if you were never sad, how would you know how great happiness feels? Sadness allows you to appreciate the beauty of contentment and joy.

DID YOU KNOW?

Treating depression makes good economic sense. For every dollar spent on direct treatment (medication or psychotherapy), it pays more than four times in increased productivity and lower health costs overall. In other words, untreated depression is expensive both for the individual and the economy.

Chapter **10**

Therapeutic Approaches

Although the rates of depression continue to increase, there are more weapons for defeating depression than ever before. Clinicians have devised new psychotherapies that have been verified as effective in treatment, as well as in preventing relapses. Medications and brain stimulation therapies continue to be refined and developed. Those with depression should feel optimistic. With persistence, recovery is possible.

What Types of Therapy Are Used to Treat Depression?

Psychotherapy for depression involves working with a therapist using psychological techniques to relieve symptoms of depression. To be successful, no matter what technique is being used, a strong therapeutic relationship must be established. That relationship should include mutual respect, kindness, and openness. Most important, you should feel safe honestly talking about your thoughts, feelings, and behaviors.

Empirically validated therapies for depression have been studied and found to be effective in treating depression. In fact, multiple studies have found them to be at least as effective as (and sometimes more effective than) medication for depression.

The following types of therapy are commonly used:

» Cognitive behavioral therapy (CBT)
» Interpersonal psychotherapy (IPT)
» Acceptance and commitment therapy (ACT)

How Does Cognitive Behavioral Therapy Work for Depression?

CBT operates on the assumption that the way people think about, perceive, and interpret events impacts the way they feel. In addition, changing the way you behave influences the way you feel. A cognitive behavioral therapist teaches people how to find flaws or distortions in thinking, challenge those distortions, and find new ways to interpret situations. They also help clients increase pleasurable activities, teach problem-solving techniques, and decrease avoidance.

What Is the Role of Interpersonal Psychotherapy in Treating Depression?

Interpersonal therapists help clients identify and modify problems in relationships past and present. Like CBT, IPT has been found to be highly effective in treating depression. Depression sometimes follows a significant disruption in important relationships. The therapist looks into areas of loss, grief, or major changes in a person's life (such as divorce or retirement). The therapeutic relationship is used to develop new ways of considering and coping with loss.

What Are the Techniques Found in Acceptance and Commitment Therapy?

ACT shares many of the techniques found in CBT. However, in ACT there is an emphasis on accepting all feelings, negative or positive, instead of trying to not have any negative feelings at all. ACT teaches that feelings are valid and shouldn't be avoided. In addition, ACT helps people uncover their most important values and live a life consistent with those values. ACT has been found to be an effective treatment for depression.

How Do Brain Stimulation Therapies Work for Depression?

Electrical or magnetic stimulation targets areas of the brain thought to be related to emotion. The purpose of stimulation is to stimulate nerve cells, rewire connections, and restore normal functioning.

Brain stimulation techniques are usually saved for cases in which traditional psychotherapy or anti-depressant medication has been unsuccessful. These stimulation techniques do relieve symptoms for some people with treatment-resistant depression. However, they're still works in progress. Further research is needed to fully validate their effectiveness.

What Is the Role of Support Groups in Managing Depression?

A *support group* is a group of people who meet in person or online to share common issues and gather to talk about their symptoms, solutions, and challenges. Support groups can be safe spaces to learn new ways to cope, to grow through the experiences of others, and to offer help to others who face the same burdens. Support groups offer hope and care. They can be wonderful additions to psychotherapy or medication treatment for depression.

TIP

Before you consider joining a support group, make sure that there are clear guidelines and expectations, that there are rules to prevent one person from monopolizing the time, and that confidentiality is maintained. Be extremely wary of a support group offering quick cures, especially when a specific product or service is promoted.

4

Living with Depression

IN THIS PART . . .

In this part, I explain how depression presents at different ages and stages of life — from childhood and adolescence through adulthood through postpartum and more — as well as how it differs in men and women. It offers strategies for managing depression in daily life and lifestyle interventions you can take — everything from diet and exercise to sleep, meditation, and more. Finally, it covers how to talk with your family and friends about your depression and find the support you need.

DID YOU KNOW?

Rates of depression peak during adolescence and young adulthood. Many people look back on those times as the most difficult and stressful of their lives. Generally, as people age, they become less depressed. And many seniors enjoy emotionally stable retirements.

Chapter **11**

Depression through the Lifespan

Although there are differences in the expression of depression throughout the lifespan, there are many similarities. Almost all people who are depressed experience the inability to find pleasure in everyday life. From the neglected baby to the senior citizen, those with depression usually appear listless. They feel life is dreary, with no promise of future happiness.

How Does Depression Manifest in Children and Adolescents?

Depression has reached close to epidemic levels among young people. The causes of depression in children and teens are the same as those for adults: genetics, trauma, isolation, and chronic stress.

Depression is rare among the very young. Rates increase throughout childhood and spike in adolescence. Children don't have a word for depression — they don't tell others that they're sad — but their behavior reflects their mood. Depressed children lack energy. They have less fun than they normally do. They withdraw from activities and from others. They may have stomachaches, reject food, get sleepy, or have trouble sleeping. They often become irritable.

TIP

If you suspect your child is depressed, gather information from other sources, such as your child's teacher, your family, or your child's caregivers. With that data, check with your child's primary care provider to rule out physical problems. Then get a mental health evaluation from a professional trained in the diagnosis of children.

Depressed teens have the same symptoms as depressed adults. Also, look for teens missing school, getting poor grades, changing friendships, and increasing irritability and moodiness.

How Does Depression Manifest in the Senior Population?

Most people are surprised to find out that emotional well-being often *increases* with age. Lots of elderly people enjoy the lessening of responsibilities, letting go of ego, and freedom of retirement. So, getting old doesn't necessarily mean getting depressed.

However, the senior years do contain many challenges that can lead to depression, such as:

» Isolation and loneliness
» Lack of purpose and meaning
» Grief and loss
» Lack of mobility
» Lack of independence

Psychotherapy and medication can help. In addition, so can some interventions that improve life, such as increased activities and more opportunities for socialization.

How Does Depression Differ in Men and Women?

Most men are socialized at an early age to believe that admitting to any kind of emotional pain is a sign of weakness. Therefore, they tend to hide sadness or depression. Instead, men are more likely to become irritable or angry. They may experience the physical signs of depression, such as changes in sleep and appetite. Although they deny depression, the rate of suicide in men is much greater than it is in women.

Women are twice as likely to suffer from symptoms of depression than men. They're more likely to be able to report negative feelings, but they also experience more trauma. Women are much more likely than men to have been physically or sexually abused (and abuse is risk factor for depression). In addition, women are more likely to be subject to poverty, chronic stress, and multiple responsibilities than men are.

How Does Depression Affect Pregnancy?

Hormonal fluctuations during pregnancy can increase the risk of depression. In addition, the stress of pregnancy itself, for some mothers, adds further fuel to the chances of developing depression.

Untreated depression in pregnant women has harmful effects on both mother and baby. For the mother, it may lead to poor immune functioning, increased risk for preterm labor and birth, increased risk for caesarean section, and higher risk of postpartum depression. The mother is also more likely to engage in substance abuse, have a poor diet, and not get enough sleep.

The baby is more likely to be born prematurely and have a lower-than-expected birth weight. They may suffer from respiratory illness and have developmental delays. In addition, babies are more likely to develop emotional and behavioral problems as they get older.

Both medication and psychotherapy are effective treatments for pregnant mothers.

What Is Postpartum Depression?

Postpartum depression is a type of major depressive disorder related to hormonal fluctuations. Depression occurs within days or weeks of giving birth. Sleep deprivation, drastic changes in life routines, and the overwhelming responsibility of having a baby are also factors contributing to depression.

TIP

A few women with postpartum depression lose touch with reality and become psychotic. They may see things that are not there, hear voices, or become paranoid. Postpartum depression that includes psychosis should be considered a medical emergency. Immediate treatment is needed to protect the life of the woman and baby.

Many women experience some mild symptoms of depression after giving birth, but they still find moments of complete happiness and joy. If your depressive symptoms don't decrease over time, become overwhelming, and result in an inability to carry out daily responsibilities, getting treatment is imperative.

DID YOU KNOW?

If you've ever been lucky enough to stand in the damp mist of a waterfall, you may have noticed a lift in spirits. Some people speculate that negative ions, produced by the waterfall, improve mood. However, negative ion machines have not been found to be beneficial in the treatment of depression. Maybe it's the combination of the negative ions and the beauty of the waterfall that works.

Chapter **12**

Daily Management Strategies

Depression impacts day-to-day life, making it difficult to cope with normal responsibilities. However, most people have to continue to meet their obligations, whether they're depressed or not. This chapter offers some ideas for managing symptoms through coping mechanisms or simple activities that can improve mood and well-being.

What Are Some Effective Coping Strategies for Depression?

When you're in the middle of a depressive episode, you probably feel like avoiding people and places. That's perfectly normal and expected. However, it isn't really the best strategy to decrease or defeat depression.

TIP

Don't expect too much, but try to find a few activities that seem tolerable to you. The idea is to increase activity. It's even better if the activities involve other people. Generally, even people with depression feel better when they're out and about. If you can't stand to make a date with some friends, go sit somewhere and people-watch.

When you're depressed, don't make any major life decisions, like selling your house, getting divorced, or quitting your job. Wait until your mood has improved with treatment or time.

Can Journaling Help with Depression?

Journaling is a very effective tool for combating depression. It's best when done as an adjunct to psychotherapy or medication for depression.

Journaling provides many benefits. It promotes self-expression and *catharsis* (the process of releasing strong emotions). It can be a tool for problem-solving. A journal can help determine what particular triggers change moods. Figuring out what causes you stress and frustration can improve coping skills.

TIP

Gratitude journals are particularly useful for increasing positive feelings. Simply write about a few things each day that you're grateful for.

Journals can either be kept private or shared with a therapist, support group, or other trusted people. Journals should be completed on a regular basis to be effective.

Does Volunteering Help Depression?

When you're depressed, your focus is inward, on yourself and your misery. Volunteering can help shift that focus from inward to outward. That simple shift can improve your mood.

Volunteering has many other benefits, too. It increases your sense of purpose and meaning, improving your self-esteem. It also promotes meaningful interactions with others, combating loneliness and isolation. In addition, volunteering has been found to increase the feel-good hormones dopamine and oxytocin.

TIP

Opportunities for volunteering can match individual interests. Some people prefer to work with animals; others distribute food. Endless choices are available. Choose a cause you care about.

How Can I Practice Acceptance to Manage Depression?

When you're depressed, you have unpleasant thoughts and feelings. For example, you may think that the future is hopeless and that you've been a failure throughout your life. These thoughts influence your feelings. In other words, negative thoughts directly lead to feeling sad and defeated.

TIP

Instead of acting defeated and sad, accept those negative thoughts as only thoughts; then let them go. That allows you to live a life despite having negative thoughts or feelings. The very act of acceptance often takes some of the power away from negative thinking and improves life satisfaction.

What Are Some Relaxation Techniques for Managing Depression?

Relaxation techniques can decrease stress and improve well-being. *Progressive muscle relaxation* is a common strategy that has been extensively studied. It has been found to be effective in pre-venting relapses, especially among those with depression and chronic pain.

TIP

The strategy involves conducting a body scan from bottom to top. During that scan, you tighten the muscles in each area for a few seconds and then release them.

Relaxation is not meant to be a stand-alone treatment for depression. It's one tool in a large tool kit.

How Can I Manage Depression at School or Work?

Most people with mild-to-moderate depression are able to function, albeit at a lower level, at school or work. The best way to manage those responsibilities is to make sure that you're getting professional treatment. Treatment will decrease symptoms and improve your ability to handle tasks.

TIP

Meanwhile, try to decrease stress as much as possible. Don't rely on your memory, which may be slightly impaired because of depression. Make to-do lists and break tasks down into small steps. If possible, take breaks and go outside for a breath of fresh air. In addition, do all that you can do to lead a healthy lifestyle (see Chapter 13).

DID YOU KNOW?

Just as lifestyle choices can decrease the risk of chronic diseases such as heart disease or diabetes, lifestyle interventions can help decrease the risk of depression. Mood is affected by diet, sleep, and particularly exercise.

Chapter **13**
Lifestyle Interventions for Depression

ifestyle medicine is a specialty in which doctors help patients improve their physical well-being by making healthy choices. Evidence indicates that there are six pillars of healthy living:

» Good nutrition
» Adequate, nourishing sleep
» Physical activity

» Stress management

» Social connections

» Avoidance of risky substances

Considerable research has documented that these behaviors prevent a large percentage of chronic diseases. This chapter looks at how they also impact mental health — in particular, depression.

Can Lifestyle Changes Help with Depression?

Committing to a healthy lifestyle helps protect against depression and it can decrease symptoms when you're depressed. Healthy eating, regular exercise, and good sleep are critical for maintaining mental health.

However, depression may make it more challenging to execute a healthy lifestyle. When you're depressed, you may not feel like moving at all, let alone participating in a regular exercise routine. Sleep is frequently disturbed during depression, and medications for sleep are rarely recommended because of potential side effects. Finally, eating healthily when your appetite has changed may seem impossible.

That's why healthy living is encouraged, but treatment for depression is recommended as a first step. With treatment and encouragement, healthy lifestyles can augment psychotherapy or medication management.

How Does Exercise Impact Depression?

If there were such a thing as a super pill, something that could make just about everything feel better, exercise would be a prime candidate. Regular exercise decreases depressive symptoms, anxiety, and chronic stress. In addition, exercise improves health, leads to longer life, provides a boost in energy and makes people feel good. When you exercise, endorphins, the feel-good hormone, are released.

Aim for about 30 minutes of exercise most days. Include endurance training (cardio), strength training (weights), and balance training.

TIP

If you have trouble fitting exercise into your life, break it down into ten-minute segments. Just about everyone has ten minutes to walk around the block, watch TV while doing squats, or do some aerobic housework. Don't let defeating thoughts get in the way of your doing something that's good for your mind and body.

Can Diet and Nutrition Affect Depression?

There are no prescribed diets for depression. However, a balanced diet is considered important for keeping the body healthy and reducing inflammation that may be associated with depression. It's important to eat lots of fruits, vegetables, and whole grains. Many health providers recommend the Mediterranean Diet, which emphasizes non-processed fresh foods as a good, nutritious way to eat.

TIP

Talk to your primary care provider to get a recommendation for a healthy diet that meets your personal needs.

What Is the Role of Sleep in Managing Depression?

Sleep problems contribute to depression, and depression contributes to sleep problems. The relationship between sleep and depression is circular.

Disturbed sleep is frequently a symptom of depression. People complain about being sleepy all the time and/or not being able to fall asleep or stay asleep. Disturbed sleep causes increased stress and anxiety, resulting in depressive symptoms.

Disturbed sleep should be considered in the overall treatment plan for depression. Cognitive behavioral therapy for insomnia (CBT-I) is an evidence-based method of improving sleep quality and efficiency.

How Does Meditation Help with Depression?

Meditation may help manage depressive symptoms, especially negative thinking. Meditation teaches you how to focus and accept all extraneous thoughts. The focus is often brought to deep breathing. During meditation practice, you observe your thoughts without judgment.

Mediation decreases stress and anxiety and can lead to a calm acceptance of problematic thoughts and feelings. Importantly, mediation decreases the constant rumination of negative thinking typical of depression. As an extra bonus, meditation also leads to better sleep.

TIP

Many meditation apps also have sleep stories, which you can use when you have trouble sleeping. The idea is to replace the loops of negative thinking that often disrupt sleep with the soothing voice, sound, or music on the app. You can search on your phone and try one for free when you're having trouble sleeping.

Can Self-Help Strategies Be Effective for Depression?

Self-help is necessary but not usually sufficient for managing depression. Many of the techniques used in cognitive behavioral therapy (CBT) are accessible in a variety of self-help formats. For people with mild depression, there are workbooks such as *Anxiety & Depression Workbook For Dummies* (Wiley), as well as multiple online options.

TIP

Although you can make progress on your own, it's best to use self-help in conjunction with a mental health professional who can act as your guide and help you access evidence-based materials.

How Can I Improve My Self-Esteem while Dealing with Depression?

Low self-esteem is a symptom of depression. If you had low self-esteem prior to becoming depressed, or if your self-esteem plummeted during a depressive episode, it's important to work on improving your self-view.

TIP

Start by taking care of yourself. Make sure you're living a healthy lifestyle with adequate rest, a nutritious diet, and plenty of exercise. Next, turn to social engagement. Start slowly with a few social activities. Don't push too hard but gently move toward doing more with people you enjoy.

Take the time to celebrate every small success, whether it's an increase in exercise or an increase in socialization. Having depression is like carrying around a 100-pound weight. You're doing a great job lifting it — keep it up!

DID YOU KNOW?

One interesting fact about online support groups is that the vast majority of members never post messages. Instead, they slink in the background, reading the other posts, just lurking. Interestingly, those who are guilty of only lurking still report gaining benefit from being part of the community.

Chapter **14**

Building a Support System

D epression damages the way you relate to others. You may avoid and withdraw from the very people you need support from. This chapter looks at managing depression in your community and with your family and friends. Part of recovery is getting help from those around you and explaining your journey through depression.

How Can I Build a Support Network for Managing Depression?

Think about the people in your life that are already supportive. Then start making plans to connect with them regularly. You don't have to tell everyone your deepest secrets, but decide who you can trust with your feelings.

If you have that person in your life already, check in with them and tell them what you need. Most people are fine with acting as a listener and an occasional advice giver. Be sure to share openly and be a good listener as well. Friendship is a two-way street.

TIP

It's perfectly okay if you don't have anyone that can play the role of listener. There are other ways to get support. Seeking out a mental health professional is a positive step toward getting help with your depression. You can also consider support groups. (See Chapter 10 for more information about treatment options.)

How Can I Talk to Loved Ones about Depression?

Family and friends may be confused by your sadness and believe that they may somehow be responsible. And some may even think that your withdrawal is a sign of rejection. So, it's usually a good idea to talk to them about your depression.

Start by deciding who to tell. Then be clear and concise. Tell them how you're feeling and educate them about depression. Explain that depression is a complex mental health illness that impacts your moods, behaviors, health, and ability to function.

If you're getting treatment, you may describe what that involves and the prognosis. Be sure to tell them that if you seem distant or distracted, it has nothing to do with your relationship.

TIP

You don't need to tell everyone in your life about your depression. Carefully consider the nature of the relationship and the possibility of an unhelpful response before you disclose personal information.

How Can Family and Friends Support Someone with Depression?

Depending on the closeness of the relationship, family or friends can offer critical support for someone with depression. People with depression need others around them to listen without judgment. They need people to tell them that they're loved and cared for.

It's hard for many depressed people to do the things that will make them feel better. Friends and family can help by engaging in social activities with them, helping them get to medical appointments, encouraging physical activity, or providing a healthy meal.

TIP

Many people express their intentions prior to attempting suicide. They may express hopelessness and complain of unbearable pain. If someone with depression expresses the wish to die or threatens suicide, take that extremely seriously. Don't hesitate — call the 988 Lifeline at 988 (or chat at https://988lifeline.org). Trained counselors will help you determine the next steps. Don't try to handle this on your own.

What Resources Are Available for People with Depression?

People with depression need information, treatment, and crisis care. For information, the National Institute of Mental Health (NIMH; www.nimh.nih.gov) provides extensive information about depression and other mental health issues.

Part of the Department of Health and Human Services, the Substance Abuse and Mental Health Services Agency (SAMHSA), has a helpline that provides referrals to support groups, treatment centers, and other resources (call 800-622-HELP).

The National Alliance for Mental Illness (NAMI) offers immediate assistance through its helpline: 800-950-6264. It also provides information about resources in the local community and access to support groups.

Local universities, health departments, and professional associations have lists of available providers and services.

For immediate crisis help 24/7, call 988.

What Role Do Online Communities Play in Depression Support?

Chapter 10 describes support groups, including online support. Peer-to-peer support communities are loosely formed groups for people who have similar problems or interests. Participants interact with others online. These groups do not necessarily have any professional monitoring or involvement.

They can provide much-needed contact with others and helpful hints, and they're available 24/7. Groups decrease isolation and provide a sense of belonging to participants.

Privacy is a concern. Although gossiping with others isn't encouraged, there are no guarantees that any personal information you share won't be shared with others. And shockingly, not everything you read online is true. Some bad actors may prey upon vulnerable people to sell, steal, or gain information. Be careful and cautious about how much information you divulge.

Online communities should never be a substitute for friends, family, and professional care.

TIP

How Can I Educate Others about Depression?

Considerable stigma surrounds mental health issues and depression. This negative perception can stall recovery. Therefore, it's important to educate people about the true nature of mental illness. Mental illness is not a sign of emotional weakness or disgrace — it's an illness, just like the flu or cancer.

If you're able, talk to people about your journey through depression. Remind them that you're still you, that depression does not define who you are as a person. Share the positive lessons that you've learned about taking care of yourself and decreasing stress in your life. Encourage others to be open about their own struggles by being an advocate for mental health.

TIP

Index

About the Author

Laura L. Smith, PhD, is an author and a clinical psychologist. She is a past president of the New Mexico Psychological Association. Laura has worked in private practice, within hospital settings, and as a consultant for schools. She has presented workshops on cognitive therapy and mental health issues to national and international audiences.

Laura is the author *of Narcissism For Dummies; Anxiety & Depression Workbook For Dummies,* 2nd Edition; *Obsessive Compulsive Disorder For Dummies,* 2nd Edition; and *Anger Management For Dummies,* 3rd Edition (all published by Wiley). She is coauthor with her late husband, Dr. Charles Elliott, of *Quitting Smoking & Vaping For Dummies; Borderline Personality Disorder For Dummies,* 2nd Edition; *Child Psychology & Development For Dummies; Seasonal Affective Disorder For Dummies;* and *Depression For Dummies,* 2nd Edition (all published by Wiley).

Dedication

The conclusion of every book project is a time for celebration and sadness. Of all of the books, this one seems like the ending of one era and the beginning of a new stage. I dedicate this book to the past and the future. I'm standing here in the present moment awaiting what comes next.

Publisher's Acknowledgments

Senior Managing Editor:
Kristie Pyles

Associate Editor:
Elizabeth Stilwell

Editor: Elizabeth Kuball

Production Editor:
Magesh Elangovan

Cover Design and Image:
Wiley

Special Help:
Carmen Krikorian